CON

ABOUT THE AUTHOR

Janet Higgins has been involved with nurse education over many years. Following graduation at London University with both a Medical Degree, MB, BS and an Intercalated Honours BSc in Physiology with Biochemistry, Janet started her career in medical research, at the Royal Free Hospital School of Medicine, in Pharmacology. It was as a lecturer at the Hospital, teaching medical students, that she was given the task of 'lecturing the nurses'. This was the start of a rewarding association with all the changes in nurse education that have happened since the 1970s to today.

Janet Higgins has held a number of senior posts, including Senior Lecturer at the University of Leicester Medical School, and Principal Lectureships at St Andrews Hospital School of Occupational Therapy (Northampton) and at Gloucestershire College of Arts and Technology. As Head of School of Health and Social Care at GlosCat she was responsible for the education of Social Workers as well as Community Nurses. Here, too, she developed new courses for Practice Nurses, working together with the local GP practices, the Family Health Service Authority, and the Education Officers of the English National Board.

Currently, Janet Higgins is the Set and Programme Leader for Health Sciences at Middlesex University. During her time at Middlesex she has been involved with the validation of both Degree and Diploma programmes leading to Professional qualifications in Nursing. She is also appointed External Examiner to the Royal College of Nursing Institute, and holds a similar appointment at Kingston University and Guildford College of Further and Higher Education, for Health Studies for qualified nurses in practice.

The focus for this book would not have occurred without Janet Higgins' partner in crime, namely Tony Higgins, Chief Executive of UCAS. As a consequence of this first-hand knowledge of the nursing education changes, national health policy changes, applications procedures, and many, many students, this book seemed inevitable.

DEDICATION

To my special husband, who puts the colour into my life, and to nursing that has formed more a central part of my life than I would have expected.

Part 1:

The Scenario

Chapter One
IMPORTANT BEGINNINGS

So you want to be a nurse!

The important thing is not to make up your mind to go into nursing practice until you are ready. People make the decision to enter nursing education at various stages in their personal or career development. Some make the decision while studying for A-levels – at school or further education college; others during the course of a university degree. Many enter nursing following work in other jobs or professions, entering as mature students (ie aged 21 or over) or with non-standard entry qualifications.

This book aims to give all those who wish to become nurses or midwives – at whatever stage – a practical approach to self-assessment, together with information and advice on the routes available.

All would-be nurses and midwives must gather sufficient recent and relevant information to make an *informed* choice, especially at this time of so much change within the National Health Service and in the number and variety of roles that can be achieved within nursing.

Getting into Nursing is written to try to make your choices easier and more effective. The aim is to assist you to make a simple check-list of questions and to consider areas for discussion. Some of the key resources and sources of information referred to in the book are listed in the bibliography, together with some useful addresses on pages 54–56.

Have you *really* identified that you wish to become a nurse or midwife, and know the reasons why you have made your choice, rather than choosing to enter one of the other caring professions allied to medicine?

Whatever you do, make absolutely sure that you have gained enough information about the various caring professions and their educational requirements to be able to make an informed choice, not

1

only for yourself but for those who will be supporting and developing your choice. You are very likely to have to talk about these matters at interview in order to gain a place in the university or college to which you have chosen to apply.

If you are uncertain of your career in health or health care, then you might be well advised to study the wider relevant subjects covered within a modular degree in Health Studies. When you have clarified your overall career plan, you could then enter your chosen clinical career with confidence that you have made the right choice. You may choose to study for a Diploma in Nursing or Diploma in Midwifery to supplement the degree that you already have achieved. The real question you have to ask yourself is, have you got enough personal resources to stand the exciting pace of change, when linked to new and demanding professional responsibilities? This applies to almost all the clinical professions but most especially to nursing and midwifery at this present time.

If you are a little further along this road of discovery, the self-analysis explored in Part 1 will give you the confidence to apply for and be successful in the next steps of 'life-long learning'. Chapters 15 and onward have been written with this in mind. Exciting professional work is constantly updated, making practice relevant to the changing needs of society. So it is with nursing, which requires you to look to the future, and ask 'what shall I be doing in five years' time, and what preparations do I need to make to get there or make my practice better?' This is true as much for those already qualified and in practice, as it is for the novice.

Chapter Two
NEW DEVELOPMENTS IN NURSING

☐ DAUGHTERS OF FLORENCE

Until only recently, very little appeared to have changed in the public's romantic image of the pretty young nurse in the starched white uniform at the bedside of the sick or injured person. In one notable London hospital, student nurses were still called Nightingales, and were trained with a thoroughness that only the 'lady with the lamp' herself could have exceeded. However, there can be no doubt that her pioneering style would have led the same lady to be at the forefront of the professional and educational developments in nursing today. One of these key educational developments, Project 2000 has had, and will have, considerable professional benefits and consequences.

☐ PROJECT 2000

Project 2000 is the name given to the recent profound change and development in nurse education, designed and implemented to meet the challenges of the 21st century. A fuller account of these exciting educational programmes is given in Chapter 3.

To understand the real relevance of these courses and to assist you in any discussion you may have with those close to you, during the application process or at interview, you should read this chapter.

The fundamental review of nursing education represented by Project 2000 was undertaken about a decade ago, spearheaded by the leaders of the profession and the nursing professional bodies. Its purpose was to bring nurses to graduate level of education, and to allow them to work alongside other health professions, notably medicine, with equivalent professional recognition, where their contribution would be appropriately recognised and rewarded. The programme was delayed by a variety of inter-professional and political issues, not the least of which was the unavailability of funding to 'free-up' unqualified nurses from work rosters in order to take time for in-depth learning, at the bedside, in the clinic, and also within university and college environments to develop knowledge, skills and attitudes to a level which reflect the demands placed upon the professional practitioner.

The English National Board for Nursing, Health Visiting and Midwifery (ENB) was largely responsible for the initiation and early implementation of these educational changes together with the colleges and institutions of higher education, including the former polytechnics (now the 'new' universities) which formed constituent partners in the process. Publications that outline many of these new developments are available from the ENB Careers Advisory Service, the address of which appears at the end of this book. One highly recommended document, *Nursing, it makes you think*, (ENB, 1994) represents many of these changes in nurse education in words and pictures, conveying high quality information in a short space of time.

Nurse education proceeding to entry to professional registration is now almost exclusively via Project 2000, by means of the Diploma of Higher Education (Dip HE) in Nursing or Midwifery Studies, currently studied primarily in colleges of health and to an increasing extent in universities and colleges of higher education, and degree studies in Nursing and Midwifery, primarily in colleges of higher education and universities, in partnership with colleges of health and clinical agencies, hospital and community trusts.

Diploma and degree qualifications both lead to professional qualification, and entry to the first part of the professional register. However, there are some differences and these largely stem from the minimum entry qualifications required for each course, generally one A-level or equivalent for the Dip HE, and two A-levels or equivalent for the degree, which satisfy the education institutes requirements. However, there are also some very important professional minimum entry requirements, which are common to both the degree and the diploma – these are clarified in Chapter 5.

The two groups of students receive monies from a different primary source in order to support their studies. Degree studies students receive their money via the usual local education authority (LEA) student maintenance grant, and the diploma student via a bursary from the Department of Health which is organised and administered by the college at which the place for study has been gained and accepted.

There is also a difference in the way in which you may apply for some of the diploma courses. Most diploma courses are available for 1996/7 entry cycle through the Nurses and Midwives Central Clearing House, NMCCH which will sometime in the near future be called the Nurses and Midwives Admissions Service (NMAS), working alongside the Universities and Colleges Admissions Service (UCAS).

The remainder of the diploma courses may be applied for through UCAS *if* they appear in the listings in the UCAS *Handbook*. At the time of going to press, the decision on which courses may be shown in which handbook was not finalised. Similarly, the arrangements between the institutions of higher education and the colleges of health are changing and developing into much closer relationships. In many cases this may mean creating a new faculty within the partner university. Whichever course you apply for, ensure you follow carefully the guidelines given to you in each of the handbooks.

The programmes of both diploma and degree studies comprise an initial period of prolonged study, the Common Foundation Programme (CFP), which develops core areas of nursing studies common to all the later branch programmes: adult, mental health, child, and mental handicap or learning disability nursing.

Midwifery is studied as an independent programme, pursuing the same educational principles, to degree and diploma (Dip HE) level within universities, colleges of higher education and colleges of health, in partnership with hospital and community care trusts.

Further specialisms, which earlier followed post-registration certificate routes, such as health visiting, district nursing, community nursing, school nurse, occupational health nurse, and practice nurse continue to form further specialist career pathways. Further details about these career choices and developments can be found in Chapter 4. If you are considering entering one of these specialisms, especially if you already hold a degree or a diploma in Nursing Studies which you may consider converting to a degree, in either Health Studies or Nursing Studies, it would be worthwhile exploring some of the postgraduate prospectuses published by individual universities and colleges.

Since this whole educational area is developing very rapidly, it is always worth checking these things out for yourself. This may be done by reference to the latest edition of *University and College Entrance* or the UCAS *Handbook* (undergraduate courses only). Postgraduate course listings are available on the ECCTIS database, and in *Graduate Courses*, a separate handbook.

☐ PROFESSIONAL COLLEAGUES

As government policy, or social policy as it is termed, has indirectly assisted the new developments in the education of nurses to meet the challenges which nurses will face in the 1990s and beyond, then it is important to mention some other professionals with whom nurses will work either directly or indirectly, and alongside whom nurses may work in educational programmes during undergraduate studies. This involves social workers and others who are involved in community care.

Social workers, like nurses, are educated to diploma, degree and postgraduate levels of education. A common area of education focus with nursing is that of learning disability, one of the branch programmes in Project 2000. The Community Care Act 1990 is slowly working its way into changing the balance of care away from institutions and into the community. This frequently seems an uphill task to all those involved. However, the primary changes have taken place, with the subsequent knock-on effects in education.

☐ PRIMARY HEALTH CARE AND PRACTICE NURSES

Before the NHS social policy changes got under way, following enactment in 1989, qualified nurses began to be employed more fully and more frequently in health centres in general practice, as practice nurses, working alongside general practitioners and other members of the primary health care team. Many, with full registration i.e. Registered General Nurses worked with full autonomy while being responsible to the general practitioner. Others, i.e. State Enrolled Nurses (SENs), could only work under supervision of a Registered General Nurse (RGN). SENs have subsequently undertaken conversion courses, validated by the English National Board, to develop their education skills to Registration Certification (see Chapter 15) and some have undertaken the three or four years of full-time study to achieve an undergraduate degree in Nursing Studies, following entry to university as mature students.

☐ CARE ASSISTANT COLLEAGUES

Unregistered individuals, care assistants or helpers may assist with hospital bedside care as part of their job specification, with defined tasks under supervision, but people in these jobs are not on recognised programmes of study leading to nursing or other professional qualifications, and are not bound by the same professional codes of conduct. Such Care assistants may undertake a National Vocational Qualification (NVQ) which by national recognition and standard may be used for progression in learning and professional development. At a later time they may wish to be considered for entry as mature students to advanced programmes of study. For entry to Nursing or Midwifery, minimum entry requirements have to be met, and these are laid out in Chapter 5.

☐ SUMMARY OF CHANGE

Nursing is at the centre of a health revolution.

First, the focus of care has changed away from illness, towards a concept of 'health and how do we maintain it'.

Second, the balance of how the government spends its money in keeping the nation well is largely changing from hospital bed to community care.

Third, the nurse is still very much the professional nurse. He or she, through professional educational developments, will be able to contribute more effectively within these changing contexts. The Code of Professional Conduct of the United Kingdom Central Council for Nursing, Midwifery and Health Visiting (UKCC) shows how relevant the clinical and professional values and standards of the profession remain today. Nursing professionals are still and always will be accountable for their own practice and responsible for the nursing needs of their patients and clients.

Chapter Three
HOW NURSING EDUCATION REFLECTS PRACTICE DEVELOPMENTS

Many of the changes now taking place in nurse education have been determined by changes in society. Life expectancy has considerably improved in the UK and the Western world, with increasing improvement in housing and diet and the development of life-preserving drugs. Meanwhile, the birth rate is declining, thus altering the demographic profile of the population. There are more older people, who are expected to place greater demands on the health care system, whether they are ill or not.

The Department of Health has set targets to improve the health of the nation by the year 2000, which has led to an increased emphasis on health education and preventative measures to improve community health, and further improve care in the community.

People as patients and clients must be cared for as individuals, and it is important for nurses and other members of the health care teams to understand a person's background and circumstances which affect his or her health in their day-to-day environment, if they are to help individuals achieve lasting health. Research has shown that those individuals who take an active role in their own care tend to get better more quickly. Listening and explaining in the caring context are therefore significant components of effective practice, enabling patients and clients to achieve this.

These major areas of focus are central to the fundamental changes which have been addressed nationally. Consequently, these are very exciting times for you to be considering entering into or developing within the nursing profession.

☐ WHAT IS PROJECT 2000?

General style and content

Project 2000 is the core programme for nurse education today, and it

8

is the fundamental pattern of education for nurses and midwives to undertake in order to register to practice. This is true whether study is towards a Diploma in Higher Education or a degree.

There are differences in the various courses offered at different institutions, but they all uphold, by their initial validations, the central themes and structure of Project 2000. Each course fulfils all the educational requirements needed in order to practice, and fulfils the practice requirements of the UKCC, by agreement with the partners at validation, including the hospital trusts and the university or college at which the course is held. Different institutions have adapted the core frameworks to reflect their strengths in staff expertise, in special interests and excellence.

It is therefore highly relevant for you to find out from university and college prospectuses, and from visits on Open Days, what the different strengths of each course are. The quality of each course has been regularly assessed by many authorities, including that which takes place at its initial validation. The major choice that you have to make is which of these courses' approaches, strengths, locations and facilities best suits your own interests, needs and aptitudes. Remember, you will be studying there for a minimum period of three years, possibly four, during initial qualification.

The core programme

The core programme is made up of two main parts: the Common Foundation Programme (CFP) and the Branch Programme (BP).

The CFP allows you to develop your knowledge of people systematically, from studies in psychology, sociology (the family and community), together with biology, or life sciences. These studies and core skills, such as communication skills, take place in parallel to those in nursing studies, both theory and early practice.

At this stage you will be supernumerary, ie over and above the workforce numbers when you are learning in a clinical setting. This clinical setting may be in the community or in a hospital placement, and is usually rotated to give you a wide variety of experience. As your experience builds you will start to apply your broad base of knowledge to an individual person in his or her circumstances. The CFP allows you to experience placements in the different branch programme areas. You will probably have already made your choice of branch programme but you may find that there is room for a change of plan.

9

Throughout the whole programme there is an increasing thread of development towards understanding effective use of human resources and health resources management, with a knowledge of financial accountability. This may sound a little difficult to comprehend at application time, but it simply means that the nurse is now a manager in the widest sense whether leading a nursing team, handling resource allocation for a unit, or developing new approaches to care.

The branch programme you undertake, which will depend on your initial choice and the availability of places, will form the second part of the Project 2000 programme, taking a further 18 months of the total three years.

The branch programmes are: Adult nursing, Mental health nursing, Learning disability nursing and Children's nursing. Although you will have been supernumerary in the earlier part of the course, you will now move on to learn through 1000 hours of rostered service, making an important contribution to the nursing team.

Some institutions may offer all the branch programmes, others may offer only two or three from the options available. Not all courses are alike. Make sure you obtain the current prospectus for the courses in question. Many of the institutions in which the courses are set are undergoing considerable reorganisation. For example, colleges of health are moving into closer association with universities and colleges of higher education. This sometimes results in the colleges of health joining the university or college of higher education, often as a new faculty.

Colleges of health, with different levels of association with universities and colleges of higher education, offer the Diploma of Higher Education. Universities and colleges of higher education generally offer degree and or diploma courses in partnership with colleges of health.

It is possible to proceed to 'top-up' the diploma course or extend studies to Honours degree via further study at Level 3 (see p. 29 for an explanation of this term), usually at university, undertaking Health Studies or Nursing Studies designed to achieve this. These studies allow the student to assess critically the subject that he or she is studying. The work may also build on the initial study of reseach method which will be part of the diploma course. The student may also have to undertake a research project, possibly within a clinical area, or on a topic related to practice.

Course locations

Colleges of health with different levels of association with Universities and Colleges of Higher Education, offer the Diploma of Higher Education. Universities and Colleges of Higher Education generally offer Degree and Diploma Studies in association with Colleges of health. Degree studies are usually sited on university and college of higher education campuses but not always. So enquire about this either on your Open Day visit or at your interview.

Course titles

Degrees are usually awarded at an Honours level, sometimes as a BA (Hons), and sometimes as a BSc (Hons), depending on the overall balance of the course content. As nursing practice is leading towards prescribing in the future, the majority of these programmes now lead to the award of BSc.

Course length

Courses tend to vary in length from three to four years full-time, and both Honours degree courses and diploma courses may take three years. You may wish to ask if the normal student term or semester applies to the course you are looking at, as you may need to use the long vacation for rostered hours of service or for observations and placement studies. Grants and bursaries are normally adjusted to support these commitments, but you need to know what the pressures may be *before* you enter a particular course, rather than once you are on it.

Entry requirements

Statutory requirements
Entry requirements may vary slightly from college to college, and from university to university, depending on the variation in overall content planned for the course, but there are certain minimum subject passes which have to be achieved, to fulfil statutory (or legal) requirements to enter nursing and, slightly differently, midwifery.

To study nursing, you must have a minimum of five subject passes at GCSE or equivalent. To study midwifery, the five subject passes must include a science subject and either English language or literature.

You must be at least 17 and a half years of age on entry, but you are allowed to apply at 16.

University and college educational requirements
The minimum entry requirement to study for Dip HE, Project 2000, is one good A-level pass or its equivalent, and four other subjects studied to GCSE pass level, or equivalent, together with many other personal attributes which can be assessed at interview or written about in the references concerning you.

The minimum entry requirements to study for Honours degree, incorporating Project 2000, is two good A-level passes, together with three other subjects to GCSE pass standard or equivalent. Other and highly important attributes will be assessed at interview together with your referees' information about these.

Mature students may enter without the formal qualifications quoted above, but need to demonstrate prior and recent learning within five subject areas, or the equivalent, thereby fulfilling the statutory or legal requirements listed. This may be achieved by completing a year studying on an Access to Nursing course, or by having previously achieved a pass in State Enrolled Nursing Certificate (valid at the discretion of the accepting institution). In addition, arrangements may be made by some colleges to allow prospective students to sit qualifying examinations, such as the UKCC DC educational test. This test was designed originally for use in the Civil Service in order to clarify, in one single examination session, the previous education attainment of applicants to the Civil Service. These tests are equivalent in value to 5 GCSE subject standard and have been adapted for use in nursing entrance assessment by the UKCC, for people who have not satisfied the statutory requirements listed previously.

Chapter Four
NEW ROLES IN NURSING: WHERE DO I SEE MYSELF IN FIVE YEARS TIME?

☐ HANDS-ON CARE

You will have discovered from Chapter 3 that it is currently possible to qualify as a nurse or a midwife either at diploma (Dip HE) or Honours degree level, studying for three, three and a half or four years depending on your course. The earliest age at which you may start is 17 and a half years, but the upper limit on age for entry is less easy to define, and depends on guidelines from each institution among other things.

Students may specialise through branch programmes to qualify in:

- Adult nursing
- Mental health nursing
- Children's nursing
- Learning disability (mental handicap) nursing.

Following initial qualification in any one of the above you may wish to specialise further, for example:

- Health visiting
- District nursing
- Community nursing
- School nursing
- Practice nursing
- Occupational health nursing
- Health education.

Diploma (Dip HE), post-diploma and postgraduate studies are available for those who are accepted on to these courses with appropriate experience and qualifications.

Shorter specialist courses, such as those concerning areas of specialist professional practice, include:

- Asthma care
- Intensive care
- Diabetic care.

Many others are listed in most of the prospectuses for the individual colleges of health, and faculties within universities and colleges. These courses are equivalent in many cases to modules within a degree programme and may possibly be credited towards a degree, by credit accumulation and transfer (CATS). (Also refer to Chapter 15.)

Tutoring and teaching roles in clinical practice may be developed by short specialist courses in this context. More substantial appointments in nurse education may be gained via an appropriate teaching qualification in higher education at masters level, following initial registration, clinical practice and specialisation.

Teaching, or managing other people's learning, may also be achieved effectively within the process of health education, which again may be studied to diploma (Dip HE), or to masters level, following earlier registration in nursing, and even in association with any of the specialisms listed above.

Almost all the roles in practice that nursing or midwifery can achieve use, to greater or lesser extent, some areas of health education. Discussion with a patient or client to enable their health improvement and its maintenance together with listening to the initial problem for that person, and his or her family or environment, centres around health education in some form.

Prescribing for nursing practice

Developments are underway for the next decade, so that there will be sufficient suitably educated and qualified nurses to take on the role of a prescribing practitioner. Current education for nursing is beginning to enlarge the area of study into pharmacology for prescribing for this purpose, in order that nurses may be able to prescribe medications in given circumstances.

Nurse-practitioner

Nurse-practitioner is the name given to an individual who in future will have undergone a more intensive education in nursing, management and treatment practice following initial qualification, and who will largely work autonomously in the care of their patients. Such nurses are already so qualified in New Zealand and the USA, and further developments in the UK are in progress, notably at institutes of advanced or postgraduate nursing studies.

☐ ONE STAGE BACK FROM THE HANDS-ON CARE?

Teaching and tutoring roles in nursing practice

You may wish to consider the area of tutoring or even becoming a lecturer in nurse education, when you have achieved your early goals in clinical practice. You may wish to pursue research in nursing by taking up a post at university. It is certainly an area of influence, either to develop practice or influence policy in health care. Most people in these roles retain their clinical, community or practitioner links in some context. It is seldom an either/or situation in professional choices. A new role is that of Lecturer–Practitioner.

The world is your oyster

You may wish to influence a range of areas which affect nursing or care directly or indirectly, but not necessarily have a direct hands-on role yourself. Nurses are now well qualified following Project 2000, to take on more senior and wider ranging roles in unit or trust management either in a care-team, unit or Trust board role. The operational management of a hospital, for example, is likely to have a Director of Quality, incorporating the work of Director of Nursing, who will also have a seat on the full Trust board.

Boards of Trust Management are responsible for community care as well as hospital care, the former in primary care, the latter largely in secondary care. Primary care, for those of you not familiar with the term, is the first point of contact for the patient or client. Treatment, or advice may be given in the primary care setting, GP practice or Community health centre. However, the patient may be referred to a hospital or specialist clinic to receive secondary care, which may for example be for an operation. Patients sometimes can be re-referred to a more central or specialist Unit. This is termed tertiary care.

Nurses are and will be more frequently involved throughout the whole structure of these new arrangements. Individually they may be responsible for assessing the health needs of the community, or managing resources to affect the care of a hospital ward, as a nursing sister.

You may also ultimately wish to safeguard the areas of practice and professional standards, or influence government policy, and social policy, by working in or with one of the professional nursing bodies such as the Royal College of Nursing, the Royal College of Midwifery, or the English Board for Nursing, Midwifery and Health Visiting, or its other national counterparts. Again, this is another branch of nursing that could be open to you in due time and with personal and professional development.

Chapter Five
WHAT DO I HAVE TO OFFER, AND WHAT SHOULD I STUDY BEFORE I APPLY?

Personal reflection should confirm that you are making an informed choice in your next steps in your life and your career path. You need to take sufficient time to make this choice. No one can tell you how much time is enough.

Do not make your decision until you have spent some considerable time gathering information, and then pause to reflect that this is what you want to do.

The next part of the process needs you to analyse whether this is a realistic choice, given that we all have strengths and weaknesses. Sometimes your passion to become a nurse may have overruled aspects of your life, your personality and your needs that demand consideration. Take time for reflection again.

It would neither be kind nor appropriate if these tough words were left out of this or any other advisory book on how to apply for nursing or another caring profession.

There are some individuals who are excluded or discouraged from entering nurse education.

For example, someone who has a history of mental illness will probably not, in the long term, be able to survive the intensive self-assessment and rigorous education process demanded by nursing. It is very important that you do not refuse to acknowledge past mental illness. You will not be of any benefit to yourself, or to your patients or clients. If you have such a history, but are well enough to undertake undergraduate studies, discuss your options with some care with a qualified careers officer or teacher working in careers guidance. You may be advised to apply for non-clinical degree studies related to social studies or health studies which may broaden your choices.

The second serious area concerns any individual with a past history of serious criminal offending. A police check for such records is performed for all applicants to nursing and social service careers which provide care to vulnerable people. If the applicant to nursing is below the age of 18 (minimum age for entrance is 17 and a half years) then a parent will normally be asked for consent.

Now for the positive side. You have no doubt got a lot to offer in terms of a career in nursing, so let's explore the potential.

Your strengths

Why not list these? They may include:

- your academic achievements
- your sense of humour
- your disposition and people skills
- your outside interests, travels, and occupations if appropriate
- the levels and length of any earlier work or experience, in caring, with older people, with children, either in your family or in a care home
- your inner strengths, eg your ability to cope with long hours, or loyalty in difficult times, etc.

There are many other personal attributes of this nature which you may like to discuss with your career advisers.

Your weaknesses

Be honest in your assessment. List your weaknesses and then work on any strategies to acknowledge them and minimise them.

If you think any are serious enough to interfere with your ability either to study at this level or with your ability to become a professional nurse, then talk this through with the careers advisers or teachers involved with career information.

☐ WHAT SHOULD I STUDY BEFORE I APPLY TO COLLEGE OR UNIVERSITY?

It is important to recognise that you will be expected to work at the level of higher education during your nursing studies whether you attend a college of health, or a faculty of health in a university or college of higher education.

If you are a mature applicant by definition, there are still some pre-requirements to be met in terms of academic qualifications before you may enter nursing studies, even though you may not need to offer the standard entry requirements.

Mature students may enter higher education without formal qualifications, but for entry to nursing need to demonstrate prior and recent learning within five subject areas or the equivalent validated study. This may be achieved by completing a year studying on an Access to Nursing course, or by having previously achieved a pass in State Enrolled Nursing Certificate (at the discretion of the accepting institution). Arrangements may be made by some colleges and institutes of higher education to allow prospective students to sit qualifying examinations equivalent to five subject areas at GCSE pass standard, such as the UKCC DC test.

Academic qualifications quoted in the colleges' or universities' prospectuses act largely as a guide in order for you to be able to succeed in your studies at the particular institution you have chosen. Many other attributes of your personality and skills will be taken into account at interview. Brian Heap, in *Degree Course Offers*, discusses various courses for nursing studies and midwifery, and notes that admission requirements for nursing vary from 20 points at A-level (ie, BCC) to 4 points (ie, EE).

However, recent research has shown that the average score on *entry* to nursing degree studies, which is not the same as on application, is 12 points (ie, CC).

These differences between admission requirements and entry scores reflects less on the quality of various courses and more on their popularity, ie more popular courses will set higher admission requirements.

They also show that A-level scores are only one indicator of aptitude for entry to professional studies at degree level. There is usually a great deal more emphasis placed on an applicant's personal qualities such as communication skills and problem-solving.

Academic qualifications other than A-levels, such as BTEC National

Diploma, level merit or above, and Advanced GNVQ possibly soon to be renamed as the Applied A-level, but not yet confirmed officially as its new title at the time of going to press, incorporating Health Sciences or Social Care, are increasingly gaining respect as students on nursing courses with these qualifications are performing well, especially in problem-solving and using their initiative in clinical placements.

It is probably self-evident that you must have a realistic appraisal of the grades or scores you are likely to achieve so that you choose your university and college courses with the likelihood of being admitted to one on which you can study happily and successfully.

Which subjects?

It is a good idea to aim for a broad base of subjects at A-level or equivalent rather than narrowing your options to similar subjects to those that you will be studying in your first year at university or college. However, some preparation for some parts of the course will no doubt help, and may be an entry requirement in some instances. Almost all the courses in most colleges are moving towards a stronger scientific emphasis, to accommodate the requirements of nursing today and in the future. Courses usually require biology, and for midwifery a science or mathematics to at least GCSE pass standard. Each prospectus should state the precise requirement. If the entry requirements are not made clear in the official prospectus, you should write to the Admissions Office, to seek formal clarification.

Your knowledge of physics and chemistry may be challenged by new subjects such as pharmacology for prescribing. Therefore, these subjects could be studied at GCSE. It is possible to study sociology and psychology to A-level. These subjects are often taken by adults returning to study. However, you will study social sciences throughout your course in Project 2000, via the topics of the individual, the family and society. Therefore, you should choose subjects for pre-entry studies which you are good at, which interest you and which you enjoy, and which suit your particular aptitudes.

You should note, however, that not all courses accept General Studies as part of their admissions criteria. Check carefully in the relevant prospectus.

Work experience

One fundamental part of your preparation before you write your application is that you should have had some experience of either working or work-shadowing in the caring sector. It is always an advantage to have had some work experience in the particular area that you have identified in your career path but, while this is desirable, it is not essential. For example, you may wish to become a community nurse, but you have not yet had the chance to spend some time attached to a nurse working in the community. However, you may have had experience of working part-time in a residential care home. This is still valid work experience. Besides, you may change your mind about your chosen career path during the course of your studies.

☐ THE WHOLE PERSON

Above all, it is important that you enjoy your pre-university/college studies, as well as your undergraduate studies. This may be the last opportunity for you to indulge your interest in subjects such as music or art.

There may be opportunities in music or art therapy later on in your career which may relate to these subjects and in which you may wish to take the option of further study and development. It would therefore be a pity if you had dropped these subjects which you enjoy, mistakenly believing that you should be concentrating only on subjects related to nursing.

Many individuals when changing from one setting to another, as in school to university, or working life to that of student, fail to build in some form of exercise or sport for pleasure or relaxation on a regular basis. As a prospective nurse or midwife, you will be seen as a role model, especially with reference to the increasing role of health education, and the policy targets for the health of the nation by the year 2000. It would be to your credit if you could demonstrate your earlier involvement in health and exercise or sport, and continue to build it into your new lifestyle.

In summary, therefore: you need to spend time on reflection, as well as time on the right set of subjects for pre-entry study and you need to spend time developing your whole person, as time invested here will be of considerable assistance to you at interview and in your future life.

Chapter Six
PERSONAL ATTRIBUTES NECESSARY FOR A CAREER AS A NURSE

The personal attributes that you need to be a successful applicant to a nursing degree or diploma, Project 2000 course are those which you need to be a nurse.

Clearly Project 2000 has been designed and put in place for nurses of the future to gain a wide education by being a full-time student in higher education, experiencing practice and relating it to underlying and related theory in nursing studies, social and life sciences.

You will be joining a profession as a student member of the team, and later, as part of that team, you will take part in rostered service during the last year of the course. Patients and members of the public will see you as a member of the nursing profession, whether you are on the first day of your course or fully qualified.

You will need to like working with people, and through this attribute be able to work more effectively with patients and clients, and also with other members of the health care team. You will need to know this for yourself, and you will need to have tested this for yourself, by working in a caring capacity for a period of time. This will demonstrate to others, your tutors and referees, that you can work effectively as part of a team to care for sick or frail people, children, or those with disabilities.

Other, less obvious attributes will become clear once you focus on the professional role that you will take up, such as the good health role model, and the ability to run your life in a health-conscious way.

Your knowledge of health education issues will be explored at interview. More importantly, you will be able to demonstrate your attitudes – to yourself, to others around you, and to those in your care.

From the start of your professional journey as a nurse, you can do no better when exploring the attitudes and aptitudes needed than to consider the wider implications of the UKCC *Code of Professional Conduct*. Clearly, these attributes of personal responsibility and the ability to reflect on personal development do not occur instantaneously. However, they are central to the whole character of the person, the student nurse or midwife, the ultimate professional and his or her professional life and practice.

The *Code of Professional Conduct* will underline for you the attributes needed at the time a student nurse enters into clinical observation and practice, latterly as part of the rostered workforce in clinical education.

In essence, it is *central* to your future as a nurse that:

- you are totally trustworthy
- people have confidence in you
- you are caring of other people
- you respect any information you may be given as confidential
- you protect the good standing of the nursing profession and society in general
- you are accountable for your actions and practice
- you safeguard the well-being of any persons within your care and you are aware of issues that concern their safety
- you can work within a team, respecting the quality of contribution from other members of that team
- you respect the customs, values and spiritual beliefs that others may hold, and their right to hold them.

Chapter Seven
HOW WILL THESE PERSONAL ATTRIBUTES BE ASSESSED?

Do not panic. This is all relatively painless, frequently fun, and sometimes pleasurably reassuring.

If you really do not have these core attributes, or embryo personality profile, it is far better to find out now than waste time and effort in trying to fit yourself into the wrong mould. It would be painful to pursue the wrong path, and it is often difficult to retrace your tracks to start in the right profession or job at a later date. But even this latter course of action is better than to stay on the wrong path.

1. Before you apply, do some informal self-assessment

If you have not already done so, and you are at the stage of considering whether nursing or midwifery may be a suitable career choice for you, there are commercial interactive software programmes available which assess you, your personality, your choices, likes, dislikes and aptitudes from a substantial series of answers you give to carefully framed questions.

Once you have identified the career direction in which you wish to proceed, and for which you are suited, you may wish to search for specific courses at specific institutions, and this may be done using ECCTIS, a government-supported computerised information service covering over 100,000 course opportunities in all universities and colleges of higher and further education in the UK.

To use ECCTIS, contact your local school, college, careers office or training access point. There are over 4000 ECCTIS access points in the UK and British Council offices worldwide. You can use the computer yourself or with the help of an adviser. ECCTIS can also provide data for credit transfer for applicants with advanced standing and also for those who are exploring career opportunities at postgraduate level (see Chapter 4).

Careers guidance at your present school or college is usually invaluable in terms of your personal assessment, as your teachers and tutors will have got to know you over a period of time, and in addition may have access to simple personality tests and questionnaires which you may like to use.

For the mature applicant, the Careers Centres found in most large towns and run by the local education authority are an excellent source of expertise and careers counselling. The advisers there will not have had the opportunity to know you over a period of time, but they will have access to a range of careers guidance material.

2. The first level of formal assessment is the self-assessment required when you complete the section about yourself, your background, aspirations and achievements on your application form. This is a very important part of the form. It is probably a good idea to make a draft – or several! – before you commit yourself on the form itself. You must complete the form in your own handwriting and, because it needs to be photocopied, you need to use a black pen.

In this section you have the opportunity to let the admissions tutor know a great deal more about you, your ideas, and your writing skills. It is particularly important that you focus on why you feel that you wish to study nursing or midwifery, why you want to enter a particular course or career path and discuss why you feel that you are suited to do this, including information about your health, and previous experience of caring.

3. The second level of formal assessment, is that done by your referees as part of the application form process, either to the NMCCH (NMAS), or to UCAS. The NMCCH requires two references, whilst UCAS requires one.

A reference in this context is not to be confused with referee, as on most occasions what is written ultimately by one person about you, and on your behalf, is usually a summary of many teachers' assessments of you and your work. The exception occurs with direct entry of mature applicants, who have not first gone through an Access to Nursing course, when a single referee writes the reference.

Where you are applying through NMCCH (NMAS), your first referee could be your teacher, careers tutor or your line-manager at work. The second referee could also be one of these or someone who knows you well. Guidance on these matters is clearly given in each of the accompanying handbooks.

The referees will have formed an opinion of you in relation to the profession you wish to join. They may know that you have spent time working in a caring capacity. It is important that they have this information about you, where and for how long. It may also be helpful for them to have a written reference from someone who knows your capabilities in this area as well. The first referee will most likely have to supply an assessment of your educational ability, and your likely potential for development in higher education. All nursing and midwifery education is now taking place either within or in close association with a university, college or higher education institute.

4. The third level of assessment is at interview. After the application, the next assessment of your personal attributes (knowledge, skills and attitudes) is at the interview.

Your general appearance, demeanour and body language will convey and possibly reinforce many of your personal attributes during conversations at the formal interview (see Chapter 15). Do not worry if you are nervous. This is a normal reaction, and admissions tutors are used to meeting and interviewing candidates who are new to the interview process, and make allowances for a few nerves in these circumstances. In addition to the formal interview, there is the informal interaction with others who are likely to have been invited for interview at the same time. You may be shown the library or other college facilities as a group, or you may be invited to have a shared discussion on a topic such as 'Should nurses wear uniforms?' Your interaction with other potential team members or course members will be relevant. In other words, very simply, how do you get on with other people, and how do they relate to you?

Another more structured method, and neither better nor worse than the other methods of observational assessment discussed previously, is for you to take a simple question-and-answer short written test, or a multiple choice test. These are known as psychometric tests, and are often used to assess a person's psychological profile and personality, and his or her potential to fulfil a particular kind of job or role. The psychometric tests are never used as a single assessment, but always as a portfolio of tests by which assessment will be finally made. They will only be used to endorse what is already known from your earlier profiles, and from your interview.

Alternatively, you may be asked to write a single 40-minute essay on a particular topic related to the caring professions, and where you may be expected to have a well-reasoned view. The topic may be a serious one, such as 'Should euthanasia be legalised for the frail older person after living years in a nursing home?' From this sort of question it would be possible for admissions tutors to pick out some of the qualities and attitudes of the applicant. This more sophisticated approach is frequently used for post-basic education entry, for example, to district nursing or community nursing.

Whatever the framework or programme of the interview day, you will normally be given an idea of what is expected of you, including any written components. You may need to bring a pen with you.

The best part of the interview day is meeting a group of like-minded people. It is even more pleasant to meet some of them again on the first day of the course.

Chapter Eight
SOME NOTES ON HIGHER EDUCATION

Higher education usually takes place within a university, but it can also take place in many other locations, such as in a college or institute of higher education. The studies accomplished there may be validated to receive a degree from a nearby university, or may stand alone as a partner with a university. A strand of higher education may also be achieved within a further education college, by a university franchising the first year of a degree course or an Access course before starting degree work. The student may then finish the second and third years of the degree at the university itself, or move to the university for the full three years of the degree after completing the Access course.

For nursing, Honours degree and diploma courses in higher education are almost exclusively placed in the new universities and colleges of higher education. The degree largely developed in the new universities (previous polytechnics) mainly because of their ability to respond quickly and sensitively to the changing professional needs of nursing, and because they have the administrative machinery to respond more swiftly than the older universities. Some notable exceptions exist, particularly Manchester University, which developed one of the earliest degrees in nursing.

A few universities run both degree and diploma courses. These are shown together in the UCAS *Handbook* and applications are made through UCAS. The majority of the Dip HE studies are currently run in colleges of health, in close association with a university or higher education institute.

Most of the diplomas in this latter group recruit through the Nurses and Midwives Central Clearing House (NMCCH). At some point in the future (possibly in time for entry in 1997/98) all courses in nursing and midwifery will be applied for through the Nurses and Midwives Admissions Service (NMAS). For more details on the admissions process, see Chapter 11.

☐ LEVELS OF STUDY

There are a number of new phrases in higher education which may require explanation.

The concept of a level of study in degree and diploma studies is a very helpful device to allow people to study in an orderly progression, ie level 1 progressing to level 2 to level 3 to graduate. It also assists people in being able to transfer the work that they have achieved in one university to another through the Credit Accumulation and Transfer System (CATS).

Level 1 is frequently subdivided into 1A, Introduction to the subject, and 1B, Foundation in the subject. Level 2 is defined as extension of knowledge, and Level 3 is defined as using analysis within these extended studies.

Level 4 denotes study at Master's level, which conveys a level of authority within the subject. Some of those of you who read for an undergraduate degree will eventually undertake Master's level studies and read for an MSc or MA in the process of life-long learning.

Nursing degrees are generally divided into defined parts of study, called modules. Many degrees in the UK are now modularised, ie they have defined blocks of study, with assessments at the end of each, instead of end-of-year examinations to assess all the areas of study.

Most universities and colleges follow the traditional academic arrangement of three 10-week terms a year. Recently, a number of universities have introduced two 15-week semesters. The number of modules you will be expected to cover each week and each term or semester will vary. You should check your course prospectus for these details.

The vacations are by no means study-free time. In nursing you will find that you may be pursuing your studies in a variety of ways, including gaining clinical experience. This allows you to fulfil the requirements of hours of study laid down by the professional bodies, notably the English National Board for Nursing, Midwifery and Health Visiting (ENB) in order to qualify and to complete the degree and diploma courses. You will also spend your vacations pursuing research or attending summer schools.

The Dip HE Project 2000 comprises Levels 1 and 2, with some work at Level 3 on some courses. Nursing degrees comprise work at levels 1, 2 and 3. Each level of study is completed by achieving 120 credits under the Credit Accumulation and Transfer System. Thus, 240 points are required for a Dip HE and 360 points are required for an Honours degree. It is possible to achieve a Dip HE Project 2000 at one institution and transfer to another to complete your study to Honours degree level. Further information on this can be found in Chapter 16.

☐ CREDIT ACCUMULATION AND TRANSFER SYSTEM (CATS)

The main idea behind CATS is to be able to transfer the 'credit', and study further at any appropriate institution.

CAT points gained are initially termed *general credit*. If you wish to gain a place on a specific named course, your CAT points have to be appropriate, and are converted into *specific credit*.

It is of no help at all if you enter a course with sufficient general credits, but without sufficient prior development and learning to be successful at the next stage. Your tutors will review what you have achieved by general credit and give you specific credit to enable you to enter your chosen course with some advanced standing.

Students who achieve 240 general credit points at Levels 1 and 2 and who successfully complete Dip HE Project 2000 may apply to have their general credits converted into specific credits and apply to continue their studies towards an Honours degree. The decision is made by the university or college of higher education.

A Registered General Nurse qualifying after 1985, and before Project 2000 was fully implemented, can offer 120 general credit points at Level 1, towards specific credit for an Honours degree course. The degree may or may not be in nursing or health studies, but could be in a wider people-based study area such as social sciences, or a single subject in one of the social sciences, such as psychology, social policy, geography or a related professional area such as human resource management. Specific credit in these circumstances is likely to be less than the general credit.

The decision for the amount of specific credit awarded and entry with advanced standing is always the responsibility of the receiving institution. Applications for undergraduate degrees is always through UCAS, whether advanced standing is granted or not. CATS is an extremely flexible system, supporting the continuing studies of the life-long learner.

Chapter Nine
THE EFFECT OF NHS REFORMS ON GETTING INTO NURSING AND MIDWIFERY

England is split into eight regions for organisational purposes. Each of these regions is responsible for planning future workforce numbers, and thereby the numbers of nurses, midwives and other health professionals who need to be educated in order to fulfil the future needs of the region. The region is largely responsible for purchasing the education and training which you and others will gain in order to qualify as a nurse or a midwife, health visitor or district nurse. The planning of provision of nurse education is achieved by partnerships with local universities, colleges of higher education and colleges of health.

You may become more aware of this process of organisation when you read the Nurses and Midwives Central Clearing House (NMCCH) application handbook and publications, than when you read the Universities and Colleges Admissions Service (UCAS) literature. This variation in approach is worth noting but should prove no barrier to gaining a place at one of the institutions to which you apply. However, it may explain some inconsistences between the two application systems.

Scotland, Wales, Northern Ireland and also the three Armed Services (Royal Navy, Army and Royal Air Force) all have further separate recruiting systems for Nurse education. The addresses to which to apply are provided in Resource Information on page 56. Neither NMCCH nor UCAS cover applications in these locations or H.M. Forces. All the specific information concerning the detail of applying through NMCCH (NMAS) and UCAS, applies only in this context. Further detailed practical information concerning other applications outside England or to the Armed Forces must be gained by writing to them direct.

The regional organisation in England is responsible for the variation in the number of places available in each region. Education and clinical training placements are limited in number, and are fixed by complex agreements at both national and local levels. Once these places are allocated, no more people may join that particular course for that intake year.

It is important to have some overview of the nature of the organisation in which you are seeking a place, and in which you are most likely to be working for a substantial part of your life. The National Health Service has recently undergone a number of reforms, undertaken largely to make best use of future resources in an environment of growing demand. It will be useful to focus on the reforms, and the new structures within the health service, in order to be able to discuss these at interview.

Health care provision is now delivered by self-governing Trusts, units of organisational activity governed by Trust Boards of Management, reflecting local as well as specialist interests. The Trusts are monitored in their activities by government offices, via the National Health Service Executive. The Trusts are responsible for their own finances and budgets, and may in future be responsible for setting their own pay structures, inside national guidelines.

The old style District and Regional Health Authorities have been reduced, in terms of both staff and powers, at the same time as the Trusts have taken up their largely self-governing roles.

The hospital Trusts, therefore, together with the universities, colleges of higher education and colleges of health, are the partners who are interested in the education and training of future staff and in choosing candidates for nursing and midwifery who will be able to develop and be developed into professional nurses and midwives of the future.

The style and content of the courses are planned by these partners, and validated by education quality control systems within the universities, monitored by the professional bodies, such as the English National Board for Nursing, Midwifery and Health Visiting (ENB).

The ENB is largely involved as an interested party in the education process of professional nursing. The United Kingdom Central Council for Nursing, Midwifery and Health Visiting (UKCC) is responsible for the quality of professional practice, and for upholding professional standards following qualification.

Obviously, although separate, these two bodies have a great deal in common, as the quality of good practice is founded on the quality of education preceding it. The ENB and the UKCC are independent of the purchasing of future employment needs but cannot be entirely separate from it in that they are the arbiters of professional quality by statute (law).

The NHS reforms can be summarised as encouraging each part of the health service, each unit, each ward or clinic, to be responsible for its own management. You may expect to find yourself in charge of such a unit one day, as a unit manager, or a ward sister. The challenges presented and met can be very rewarding, following personal and professional education and development to meet the education and training needs of that appointment.

Part 2:

The Essential Preparations for a Successful Outcome

Chapter Ten
OK, SO I STILL WANT TO BE A NURSE

The essential preparations for a successful outcome to your application must include a check-up on your current educational position, together with an honest assessment of your personal development. If you find that you do not meet the strict criteria of the entry requirements, then you may need to go a stage or two back and concentrate on achieving these before you make an application, otherwise you will clearly be disappointed by your lack of success. This could also mean that you may also find yourself on the wrong course or in the wrong professional role.

☐ CHECKLIST FOR APPLICATION CRITERIA

1. Will you be over 17 and a half years of age on entry to university, college of higher education or college of health?

2. Do you really know that you can work with people?

3. Have you gained evidence both for yourself and others that you can work in the care sector caring for other people?

4. Is it really nursing that interests you, or have you not yet made up your mind as to your final career path, or your professional role in caring?

5. Will you be able to study full-time for at least three years, within higher education (for diploma and degree courses within Project 2000)?

6. Do you fulfil the minimum entry requirements for nursing or midwifery studies at the time of your application? These minimum requirements are different for midwifery compared with nursing. Check these again.

7. Do you have a criminal record? This will be checked on receipt of your application.

8. Are you in good health, and do you expect to remain so?

9. Do you understand the criteria to be met by the UKCC *Code of Professional Conduct*?

10. Can you live by these criteria for the remainder of your professional life?

Chapter Eleven
APPLYING THROUGH THE SYSTEMS

If you have successfully completed the checklist in Chapter 10, and have undertaken a long period of reflection, you will now have a clear idea that a career in nursing or midwifery is a real possibility rather than a hope. Your next steps are to pursue your goal with purpose.

You need to clarify your approaches to the two separate application systems, which may have merged by the time of entry to courses in 1997/98.

At present, you may apply through UCAS, for all undergraduate degrees in nursing and midwifery, Project 2000, and for some diplomas (Dip HE) Project 2000. There is one application cycle per year for entry to the institution of higher education in late September. For Dip HEs in nursing and midwifery, there is one application cycle through NMCCH per year, deadline May, and two entry programmes in August and February.

Decisions will shortly be taken as to how to bring these two systems together for nursing and midwifery education application procedures, probably for the 1997 entry cycle. Detailed changes are yet to be finalised, and will need clarification by you if you are applying after the 1996/7 entry cycle. Contact information is available at the back of this book.

☐ APPLYING THROUGH NMCCH

NMCCH admits the majority of nursing and midwifery applicants. There are three times as many applicants as entrants.

There are eight National Health Service Executive regions in England with about 162 institutions offering Diploma (Dip HE) education programmes via the NMCCH.

The large number of institutions together with the large number of applicants would lead to chaos if there was no central coordination of which place is offered and to whom. With the NMCCH application you can choose up to four nursing or midwifery education institutions, using their codes from the NMCCH *Handbook* when you complete the application form. You may only complete one application form for each application year/cycle. You also enter a choice of 'Preferred Region', as if at a later date a place becomes available, and you are still waiting to gain a place, then a better match for a likely candidate can be made.

☐ APPLYING THROUGH UCAS

There are about 50 universities and colleges of higher education offering undergraduate degree courses in nursing, and about 15 similar institutions offering degrees in midwifery. All of these are listed in the UCAS *Handbook*.

You may make up to six choices of institution or course from the codes listed in the *Handbook*, using one form per application year, including 'Clearing', the final round of places to be gained for the year's cycle. There are some minor paperwork transactions to be completed if you are still looking for a place during Clearing, but they all follow on from your initial and only application.

When your application has been received and processed, you will start to receive replies from your chosen institutions. Assuming you have been offered more than one place, you should accept one offer as your firm choice (Cf) and another, requiring lower grades or point scores as your insurance choice (Ci). You should decline any remaining offers.

There are many well-informed and well-written short texts offering advice on what you should consider when you make these decisions. Your choices are final and therefore very important. A short list of recommended texts are listed at the end of this book.

☐ CLEARING

By applying through NMCCH and UCAS, it is possible to apply to a total of ten institutions. This gives you a good chance of gaining a place somewhere, providing you meet the minimum entry requirements. However, if you miss out in the first and subsequent rounds of the cycle of gaining a place for the year in which the application was made, then the net of institutions becomes much wider in the process known as 'Clearing', which occurs just before the courses start. This is a means by which the final places are filled.

In the NMCCH system, if your form has been sent round to the institutions of your choice, in order of your preference, and you have not been called for interview and offered a place, then the Preferred Region indicator will operate in order to match your application with a place in higher education for diploma studies.

In the UCAS system, applicants are issued with Clearing C-forms in order to take part in Clearing and to secure a place on offer. This has been termed an unofficial Passport to gain and confirm a place on your behalf, without which the place cannot be secured.

If you find that you do not want to accept your original choice of Cf or Ci institution, then you must formally reject the offers you have received and take your chance on entering Clearing. You cannot enter Clearing unless you have rejected all offers or you hold no offers whatever at that time. You will then be issued with a C-form.

Chapter Twelve
CHOOSING YOUR COLLEGE OR UNIVERSITY, AND GETTING CHOSEN

☐ CHOOSING

Nursing and midwifery are no longer in the unusual position that individuals are educated to professional status, and develop to professional practice in isolation, separate from other professional groups. Now, all the benefits and resources available to other higher education entrants are available to those entering nursing, midwifery and the many career pathways that develop from initial qualification and registration. As a consequence, all the information that is available for others going into higher education is available and can be made to work for you, in addition to all the specialist information that you have concerning the education processes for nursing and midwifery.

Getting into University and College, 1994, (see p. 54) is a short and highly relevant guide and checklist which allows you to take charge of your own choices leading to an undergraduate degree course. Detail is given as to how you may make your choice; make a timetable to achieve a good outcome; consider criteria in choosing among differing courses; and the choice of institution, together with choice of location, city, suburban or rural settings. Similarly, a great deal of unofficial information is given by Brian Heap in *Degree Course Offers*, updated annually. These key references are available in most libraries or careers offices.

For information on which to base choices for the course and the institution for entry to Dip HE courses in nursing and midwifery, the *Applicant Handbook* from the NMCCH is the major source.

Once you have made a shortlist of courses and locations, write to the relevant institutions and obtain any promotional literature, together with the prospectus, including the alternative prospectus, produced by the Students Union for a different view of the institution. Remember any promotional material produced by the institution is designed to show it in the most favourable light. When your shortlist is reduced to about six, make every effort to visit it on Open Day for a closer view.

☐ GETTING CHOSEN

Your first formal contact with the institution to which you have applied will be via your application form, and this must be filled in correctly. Details on getting it right and getting it in by the stated deadlines are given in the *Applicant Handbook* for the NMCCH, UCAS *Handbook* and *How to Complete Your UCAS Form for 1997 Entry.*

It may seem self evident but to be successful in your application for a place to study nursing or midwifery, your application form must be completed *accurately* and posted *in time* to reach NMCCH or UCAS by the deadline.

Make sure your referees know what is expected of them, and what areas they should cover on your behalf. This is a reference to support your entry to higher education, not a job application. Sometimes, referees in the workplace do not understand this difference, nor have knowledge of you in this capacity. It is your responsibility to check this through, and not the responsibility of the receiving institution to have to write for a fuller reference if the first one does not give enough appropriate information.

What happens if several institutions make you an offer?
If this is the case, hard choices have to be made, and by a given deadline or all offers may go by default.

For NMCCH, and for 1996 entry only, you may hold a single Firm Offer, or a Provisional Offer, for diplomas in nursing and midwifery.

The *Applicant Handbook* shows clearly how the NMCCH application procedure works through your four choices. When you firmly accept an offer, you must at the same time reject all others. As the process has been operating in order of your preferences, it is not likely that you will hold more than one offer at the same time. You must respond to the offer within 14 days. This means that you must have done your homework about the institution and its location in the spring or summer vacations a year earlier. It is important for a happy and successful time at your institution that you have thought carefully about living there for the next 3–4 years.

For UCAS, choose your Firm Offer, Cf, and your Insurance Offer, Ci, by reference to as much information as you have obtained earlier, including visits to the town or city, and information gathered on Open Days. The Firm Offer is one you will hold until the conditions of the offer are met, or not. The Insurance Offer is held just in case you do not make the grade requirements of your Firm Offer. However, the Insurance Offer must also be a realistic choice, a course or institution that you will be willing to accept if you cannot meet the requirements of your Firm Offer.

Chapter Thirteen
IF YOU DON'T AT FIRST SUCCEED . . .

If you are not successful in your first round of applications, either through NMCCH or UCAS, and are still keen to get on a course try Clearing. There are two main publications to assist your progress through Clearing.

The first is *Clearing the way*, by T. Higgins (published by Trotman) which gives an information path and simple guide to assist those working their way through the UCAS clearing process, attempting to find a place on an undergraduate programme in nursing or midwifery in the few weeks before the start of the term or semester. The original application form generates an automatic clearing entry form, C-form, when the applicant has not yet gained a place and holds no offers in the UCAS system.

The first thing to remember is not to panic and not to make rash, unconsidered decisions.

The second thing to remember is that you must be realistic. Most people who are qualified will eventually find a place within the system, but not necessarily studying the subject they first wished. This may mean that you may have to start by studying for a diploma and then work towards getting a degree.

This leads to the second publication, *The Applicant Handbook* published by NMCCH, which outlines very precisely the process for those already within the NMCHH system, applying for diplomas in nursing and midwifery.

Chapter Fourteen
I AM A REGISTERED NURSE AND
WISH TO STUDY FOR A DEGREE

The date of your registration is significant in this context, and in the next stages of your learning development. If you registered and qualified as a nurse or midwife after 1985 in the UK, then you have gained 120 general credit points at Level 1. How these are translated into specific credits depends on the receiving institution at which you wish to study, and the subject areas of the degree that you wish to enrol upon. The likelihood is that you may need to study for all of Levels 2 and 3, for 240 points, plus an extra module at level 1b to support your work in any new area.

It is a matter of matching your past achievements to the degree programme you wish to enrol on, in order for you to be successful.

All full-time undergraduate degree applications are handled by UCAS, even though you may wish only to apply to a single institution, and for a single course, and the tutors have given you a verbal offer of a place. You must send for or obtain a current UCAS form, follow all the instructions in detail, including referees, fee and timing of responses. You might even wish to exercise the remainder of your choice of six options of institutions.

Although all initial nursing and midwifery degrees and diplomas are full-time, top-up or post-registration courses may be studied part-time. Part-time applicants for degree courses do not at the present time have to apply via UCAS, but can apply directly to the Institution. In this event there is usually no application fee.

As you are already registered to practice as a nurse or midwife, then your choice of degree could easily be more wide-ranging than nursing and midwifery. You could study Health Studies, either alone or with another closely allied subject, such as Psychology, Sociology, Women's Studies, Third World Studies, or Education Studies. This may open up more career paths, and wider options in the NHS, or other agencies, working across the world.

If you have registered before 1985, then you may apply for the same range of degree options but you may not gain any general or specific credit in the programme. You will enter at Level 1, and proceed through the degree programme in the usual way. Your application should be made through UCAS for a full-time course and direct to the university or college for part-time study. Full-time study qualifies for a local education authority award, but there is no such grant support for part-time study, whether you are in work or unemployed.

If you are a mature applicant, defined as an applicant over 21 years, with work or life experiences over a period of time, then you may need a more targeted form of careers guidance in order to maximise your chances of gaining a place at university or college. Motivated mature students up to the age of 40 usually achieve better degree results than their younger standard-entry counterparts. Recommended reading to assist the mature applicant is listed at the end of this book.

Part 3:

Next Steps in Life-long Learning

Chapter Fifteen
PERSONAL RECORD OF EDUCATION AND PROFESSIONAL PRACTICE (PREPP)

Many nurses and midwives already in practice do not fit into any of the earlier categories of students or prospective students in life-long-learning. Yet they still need to appraise what learning they have already achieved, and to have it recognised formally, in order to build on it and to improve their clinical practice.

Clearly nursing and midwifery, like many other professions, need to respond to major changes taking place in practice, and in clinical developments and settings, as well as keep pace with major social changes in health-related matters. The English National Board and the UK Central Council for Nursing, Midwifery and Health Visiting have initiated and developed a framework for collating and presenting a Personal Record of Education and Professional Practice (PREPP) not unlike the student Record of Achievement used in schools.

The PREPP may be used in a similar manner as the Record of Achievement. Records of continuing education for life-long learning will be a regular feature of job applications and personal profiles. Evidence of learning achievement allows individuals to be credited with what they have done at all levels of their work and practice.

Chapter Sixteen
I HAVE A DIPLOMA IN NURSING AND WISH TO STUDY FOR A DEGREE

The Diploma in Higher Education forms the main route for the education of nurses and midwives to initial registration. It forms the first two levels of the undergraduate degree, thus representing 240 general credit points for transfer. If the holder of a diploma in nursing or midwifery wishes to study for a degree, he or she should apply via UCAS if study is to be full-time. Application for part-time top-up degree programmes should be made direct to the receiving institution.

A local education authority (LEA) grant may be available for study and living support, if the study is full-time, and you have not previously held an LEA grant. There is no LEA grant for part-time study, whether the person is unemployed or in work. Most applicants who study part-time on full-time degree programmes are supported to varying levels by the Trusts or others who employ them.

The variety of degree subject areas for which you may apply are wider than those in nursing and midwifery, and are described earlier for the person who has a post-1985 RGN. Joint Honours degrees widen your options and your job opportunities. Modular science-based subjects, such as pharmacology or epidemiology, may enhance your development to assist the changes taking place in nursing practice for the future. These modules are often part of a modular science-based degree in Health Studies, forming an Honours BSc degree.

Chapter Seventeen
THE NATIONAL NURSING BODIES

The English National Board for Nursing, Midwifery and Health Visiting (ENB) is largely responsible for the quality of education of nurses, midwives and health visitors in England today. It is centrally involved in the understanding that the quality of education leads to the quality of care and uses this phrase for its logo. There are similar boards for Wales, Northern Ireland and Scotland, defined and put in place by government statute. The addresses of all these boards are available in the last chapter containing resource information.

Similarly, the national statutory body responsible for practice quality is the United Kingdom Central Council for Nursing, Midwifery and Health Visiting (UKCC). This body is responsible for developing and monitoring the *Code of Professional Conduct* for practising nurses and midwives. This Code provides the focus for exploring the personal qualities that are needed for practice as a nurse or midwife. The UKCC is also responsible for disciplinary procedures if quality of practice is not adhered to. Nurses can be removed from the Register and from practice. Education and practice standards are closely interwoven, and, as a consequence, these two bodies may become linked even closer in future.

The other major player in the national forum for nursing is the Royal College of Nursing. It has two main arms of operation: one arm functions largely as the political voice of nursing, holding talks with government and other national agencies, representing its members when and where necessary; the other arm is that of an institute of higher education and of advanced nursing education, as at the Royal College of Nursing Institute, where undergraduate-level 3 degree and postgraduate studies are achieved, mostly for post-registration nurses and midwives who have already achieved registration through earlier studies and clinical practice.

All three of these national bodies have been changing swiftly and dramatically in response to current nursing professional health changes. They are the leading bodies which are responsible for taking nursing forward to the 21st century.

Chapter Eighteen
RESOURCE INFORMATION AND CONTACT DATA

Baggot R, 1994, *Health and Health Care in Britain*, Macmillan

Boehm K & Lees-Spalding J, Edits, 1996, *The Student Book*, Macmillan

Department of Health and Central Office of Information, 1994, *Nursing: it Makes you Think*, Health Service Careers, HMSO

Heap B, 1996, *The Complete Degree Course Offers*, annual, Trotman

Higgins T, 1995, *Clearing the Way*, Trotman

Higgins T, *How to Complete your UCAS Form for 1997 Entry*, Trotman

Institute of Advanced Nursing Studies, (Royal College of Nursing Institute), 1993, *ENB Higher Award Information Pack*, RCN

Jacobson B, et al (1991), *The Nation's Health*, King Edward's Hospital Fund for London

NMCCH, *The Applicant Handbook 1995-6*, NMCCH

Thorley H, 1994, *Getting into University and College*, Trotman

UCAS, 1995, *Advice for Schools, Colleges and Careers Offices, 1996 Entry*, UCAS

UCAS, 1996, *A Parents Guide to Higher Education*, UCAS

UCAS, 1996, *A Mature Students Guide to Higher Education*, UCAS

UKCC, *Code of Professional Conduct*

UCAS, *University and College Entrance: the Official Guide*, annual, UCAS

Williams J, 1995, *Revival of the Fittest, Nurse Leadership*, Health Service Journal, 24 August issue

☐ USEFUL ADDRESSES

Department for Education and Employment, Publication Centre, PO Box 2193, London E15 2EU

ECCTIS, Oriel House, Oriel Road, Cheltenham GL50 IXP

English National Board for Nursing, Midwifery and Health Visiting, (ENB), Victory House, 170 Tottenham Court Road, London W1A 0XA

Nurses and Midwives Central Clearing House (NMCCH), PO Box 9017, London W1A 0XA

Trotman Careers Guidance and Education Resources, 12 Hill Rise, Richmond, Surrey TW10 6UA

United Kingdom Central Council for Nursing, Midwifery and Health Visiting (UKCC), 23 Portland Place, London W1N 3AF

Universities and Colleges Admissions Service (UCAS), Fulton House, Jessop Avenue, Cheltenham, Gloucestershire GL50 3SH (Application materials, including the UCAS *Handbook 1996 Entry* from PO Box 28, Cheltenham, Gloucestershire)

WALES
Careers Information
Welsh National Board for Nursing, Midwifery & Health Visiting, Floor 13, Pearl Assurance House, Greyfriars Road, Cardiff CF1 3AG Tel: 01222 395535

SCOTLAND
CATCH
PO Box 21, Edinburgh EH2 1NT

NORTHERN IRELAND

Recruitment Officer

National Board for Nursing, Midwifery & Health Visiting for Northern Ireland, RAC House, 79 Chichester Street, Belfast BT1 4JE Tel: 01232 238152

ARMED SERVICES

Royal Navy

You are advised to contact your nearest Navy and Marines Recruiting Office (see local telephone directory).

Army

Lt Col L J Murray, Regimental HQ, QARANC, Keogh Barracks, Ashvale, Aldershot, Hampshire GU12 5RQ
Tel: 01252 340298

Royal Air Force

MD & NSLO, D of R&S, PO Box 1000, Cranwell, Sleaford, Lincolnshire NG34 8GZ